THE METABOLISM RESET DIET FOR ALL

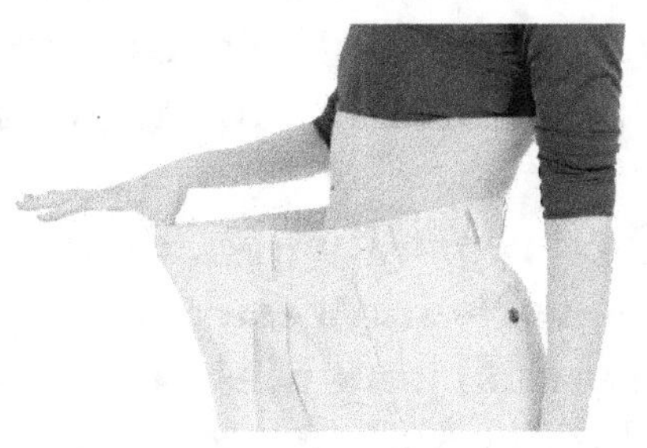

Reduce body fat,improve your brain health and aid weight loss

Dr. RUTH T. Todd

TABLE OF CONTENTS

Introduction

I used to be a lot heavier, and I hate to acknowledge it. and it was very difficult. People would ogle me and make derogatory remarks about my girth everywhere I went. Finding clothes that suited me was difficult, and I frequently felt uncomfortable.

But later, I made the decision to take charge of my health. I began eating well and working out frequently. Though initially challenging, I soon noticed that I had more energy and felt better all around.

I began to lose weight as long as I continued my healthy habits. I initially saw a slow improvement, but ultimately I began to notice a noticeable difference. Previously too-tight clothing was now too-big,

and individuals began to Observe the alterations to my look.

But more significantly, I began to feel happier and more confident. I was pleased with the advancement I had made and no longer felt self-conscious about my appearance. The trip had its ups and downs, but in the end it was all worthwhile.

Understanding your metabolism is crucial for maintaining good health and achieving your weight loss or fitness goals. Your metabolism is the process by which your body converts the food you eat into energy that powers all of your bodily functions, from breathing and digestion to exercise and movement.

A guide to your metabolism can help you understand how your metabolism works, what factors influence it, and how you can overcome it for better health and wellbeing.

This book will cover the basics of metabolism, including the different types of metabolism, the factors that influence metabolism, and how you can adjust your diet and lifestyle to improve metabolic function. You will learn about the role of macronutrients, such as carbohydrates, proteins, and fats, in metabolism, as well as the importance of micronutrients like vitamins and minerals. You will also discover how exercise, sleep, and stress can affect your metabolism and what you can do to improve these factors.

This manual will also explore some common myths and misconceptions about metabolism, such as the idea that metabolism slows down with age and that certain foods or supplements can boost metabolism significantly. Finally, you will find practical tips and strategies for optimising your metabolism, such as eating a balanced diet, staying hydrated, and getting regular exercise.

Whether you're looking to lose weight, build muscle, or simply improve your overall health, understanding your metabolism is a critical first step. By following the guidance in this book to your metabolism, you can take control of your health and wellbeing and achieve your goals.

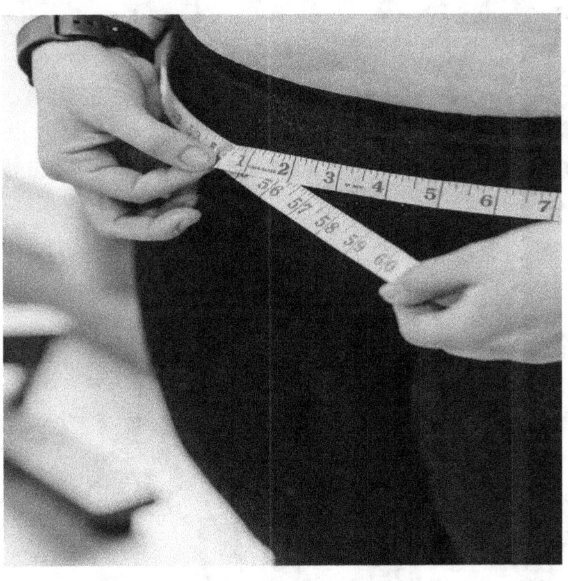

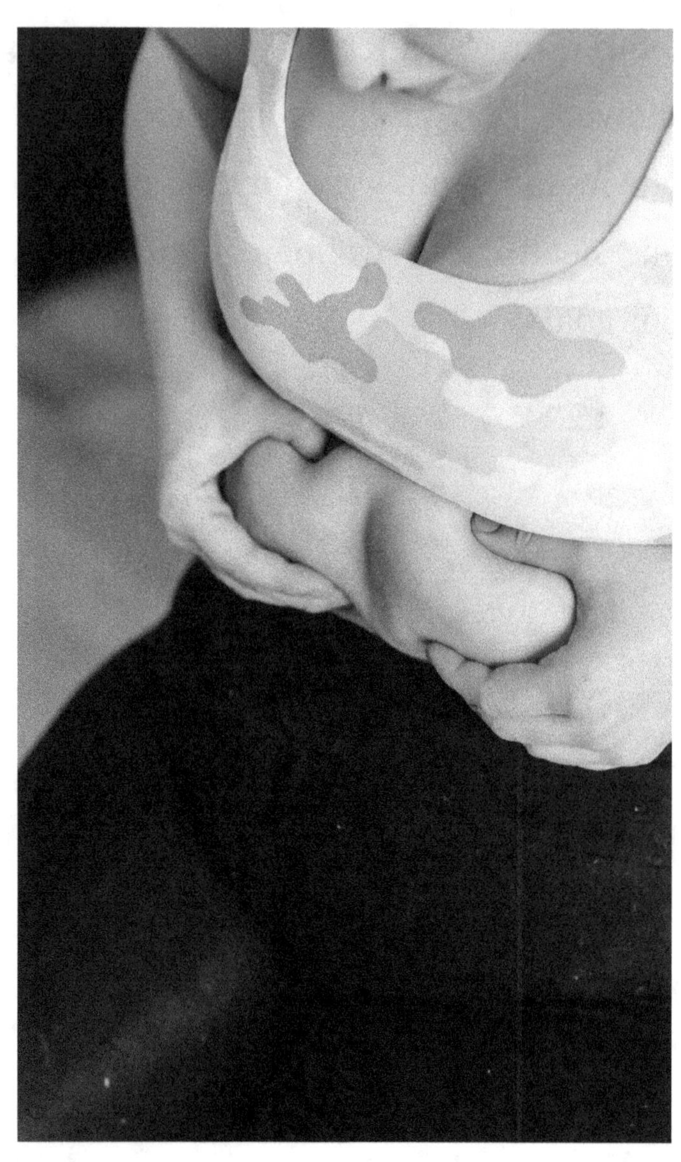

Chapter 1: Explanation of metabolism

The collection of chemical reactions that take place within an organism to sustain existence is known as metabolism. It entails a number of biochemical processes that break down food into energy, create and maintain cells and tissues, and get rid of waste. Fundamentally, metabolism is the process by which the body converts substances into the building blocks required for cellular development, maintenance, and energy synthesis. It involves the conversion of food into energy and the building and repair of tissues. Metabolism can be broken down into two main categories:

Catabolism

Anabolism.

Catabolism is the process of breaking down larger molecules into smaller ones, such as the breakdown of carbohydrates, fats, and proteins into their individual building blocks. This process releases energy, which is used to power cellular processes and physical activity.

Anabolism, on the other hand, is the process of building larger molecules from smaller ones. This includes the synthesis of proteins, carbohydrates, and fats from their individual building blocks.

Anabolism requires energy to fuel the synthesis of these larger molecules.

The rate at which your body metabolises food and converts it into energy is influenced by a variety of factors, including genetics, age, sex, body size, and physical activity level. Some people may have a faster metabolism, which means they burn calories more quickly and have an easier time maintaining a healthy weight. Others may have a slower metabolism, which means they burn calories more slowly and may be more prone to weight gain.

Factors that can influence metabolism include diet, exercise, and sleep. A balanced diet that includes a variety of nutrient-rich foods can help support a healthy metabolism, while regular exercise can help boost metabolism and burn calories. Getting enough sleep is also important, as sleep deprivation can disrupt metabolism and lead to weight gain.

Overall, maintaining a healthy metabolism is important for maintaining a healthy weight and overall health.

Its importance in weight loss and management

The metabolism is essential for managing and losing weight. The term "metabolism" describes the molecular reactions that take place inside the body to transform food into energy. Your metabolism, which is primarily influenced by factors like age, gender, genetics, and lifestyle, determines how quickly your body burns calories.

To lose weight, you must generate a calorie deficit, which is done by consuming fewer calories than you expend. Even when you're not busy, raising your metabolism can help you burn more calories.

In other words, you can consume the same amount of food and still lose weight, or you can eat more food without gaining weight.

There are a number of natural methods to increase your metabolism, including:

Building lean muscle mass through strength training:
Lean muscle mass can be increased through strength training because it consumes more calories than fat. This increases metabolism.

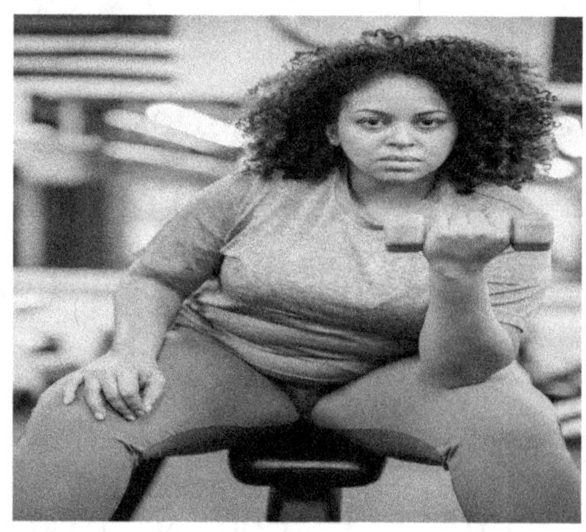

Consuming enough protein: Protein needs more energy to digest than other nutrients due to its high thermic effect. Your digestion may be boosted as a result

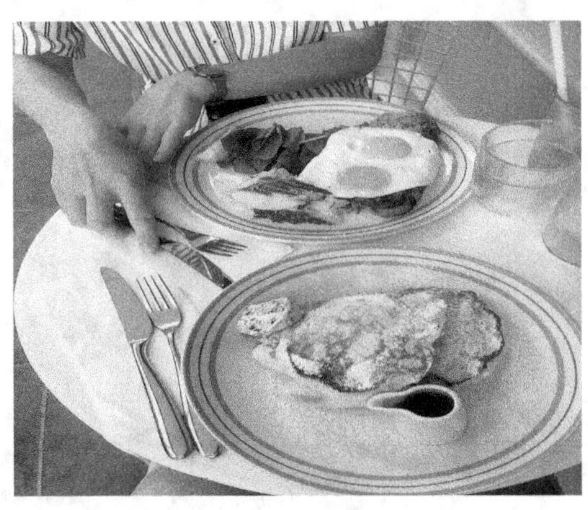

Drinking enough water: Getting enough water to consume throughout the day is important because dehydration can slow down your metabolism.

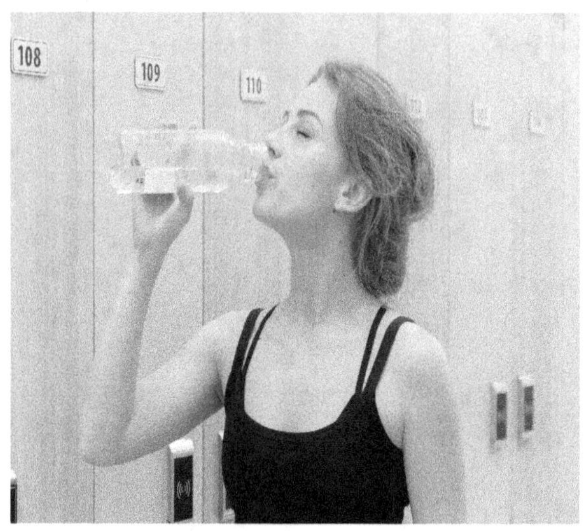

Eating enough food:

Your body will try to preserve energy if you eat too few calories, which will cause your metabolism to slow down.

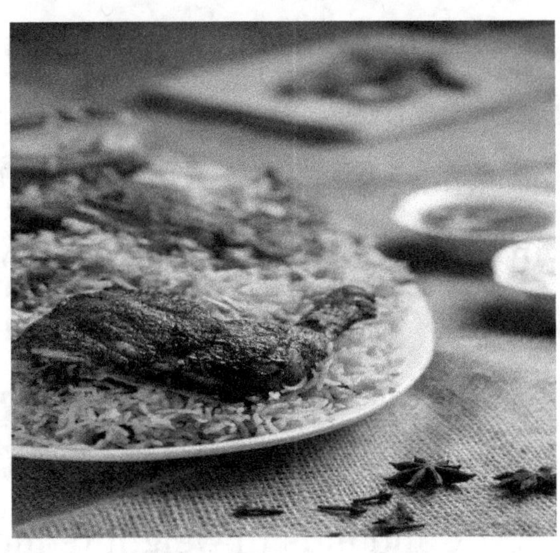

Aim for 7-8 hours of slumber per night because insufficient sleep can interfere with hormones that control metabolism. When the body burns more calories than it takes in, weight loss happens. This can be done by increasing metabolism-boosting physical exercise or decreasing calorie intake. BMR can be increased and weight loss can be aided by eating a balanced meal high in protein and fibre and exercising frequently.

Exercise and physical activity can boost BMR in addition to boosting the body's metabolism throughout and after exercise. Lean muscle mass is created and maintained through exercise, which raises BMR and aids in weight reduction. Exercises that increase metabolism and burn calories, such as strength training and high-intensity interval training (HIIT), are especially effective.

In summary, metabolism is crucial for both weight reduction and weight management. a healthy diet, consistent activity,and promotes weight loss.

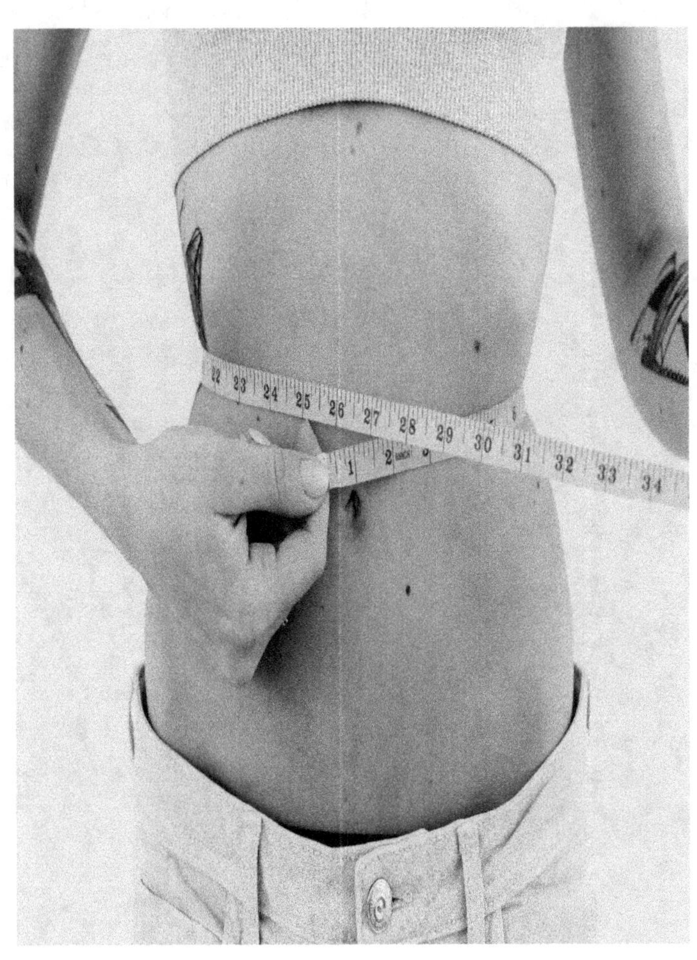

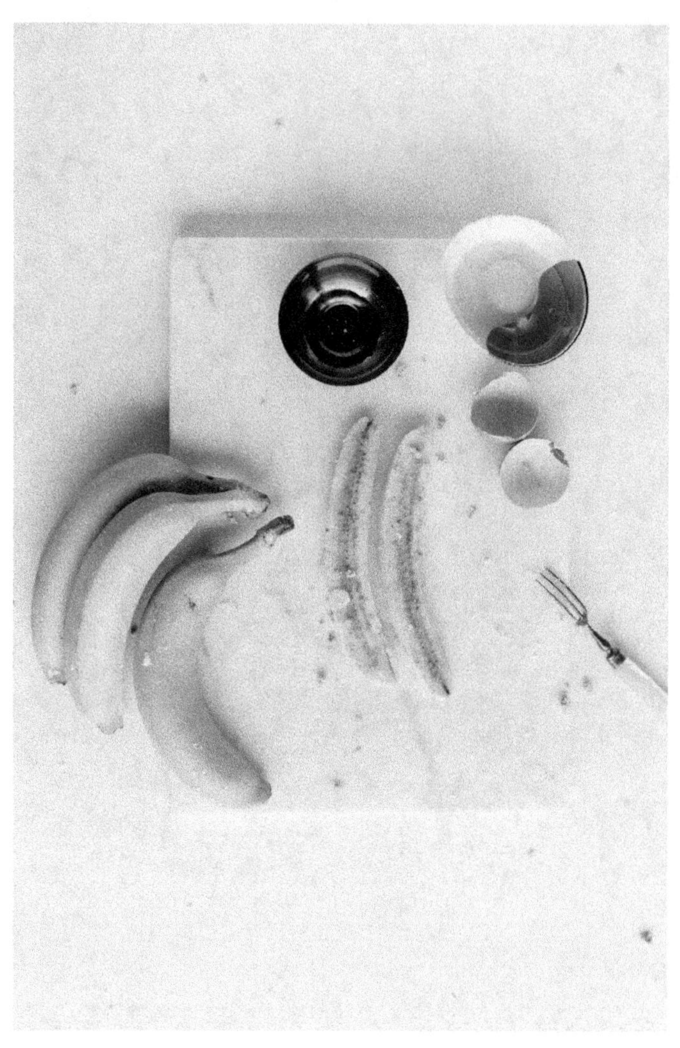

Chapter 2: Foods to Include

Foods to include in the metabolism reset diet include:

- lean proteins like chicken fish, and tofu,
- carbohydrates like whole grains,
- healthy fats like nuts and avocado,
- fruits, and vegetables
- plenty of water to stay hydrated.
- Probiotic-rich foods

These foods are high in nutrients, fibre and water, which help to keep
the body feeling full and satisfied while also promoting good digestion.

In addition to a healthy diet, it also emphasises regular exercise.

Overall, the metabolism reset diet is a balanced and sustainable approach to weight loss and management that focuses on boosting metabolism through a healthy diet and exercise. By including a variety of nutrient-dense foods and regular physical activity, this diet can help individuals achieve their weight loss goals while also promoting overall health and well-being.

Including these foods in your diet can help provide a range of nutrients and health benefits.

Lean proteins

Lean proteins like chicken, fish, lean beef, and tofu can still help boost metabolism.

When you consume protein, your body has to work harder to digest and absorb it compared to carbohydrates and fats. This process is called the thermic effect of food (TEF) and it increases your metabolic rate for several hours after a meal.

Additionally, consuming protein can help build and maintain muscle mass, which is also important for maintaining a healthy metabolism.

Therefore, including lean proteins as part of a balanced diet can be beneficial for maintaining a healthy metabolism.

Carbohydrates

Due to their slower rate of digestion and release of glucose into the bloodstream, low glycemic index (GI) carbohydrates like sweet potatoes, quinoa, and brown rice can be advantageous for metabolism. This serves to stabilise blood sugar levels and prevents energy peaks and crashes. For those who have diabetes or insulin intolerance, this may be especially beneficial.

When we eat carbs, they are converted into glucose, which the body uses as fuel. Although some carbohydrates are metabolised and absorbed more rapidly than others, this causes a sharp rise in blood sugar levels. This may cause the hormone insulin to be released, which aids in moving blood glucose into the cells for use as fuel. But over time, frequent blood sugar increases and insulin levels can cause metabolic problems like insulin intolerance.

Contrarily, low GI carbohydrates take longer to digest and assimilate, which prevents sudden spikes in blood sugar levels. This may support improved digestive health by regulating insulin levels. These carbohydrates can also offer a consistent source of energy that can support physical exertion and exercise, both of which are critical for healthy metabolism. Furthermore, they frequently have a higher nutrient density.

Healthy fats

Healthy fats, such as those found in avocados, nuts, and olive oil, can help lower cholesterol levels and reduce inflammation in the body. They are also important for brain and heart health. Consuming healthy fats like nuts and avocado can have a positive impact on metabolism.

Firstly, these foods are a good source of monounsaturated and polyunsaturated fats, which are considered healthy fats. These fats are known to improve cholesterol levels, lower blood pressure, and reduce the risk of heart disease.

Secondly, consuming healthy fats can increase satiety and reduce cravings, leading to a reduction in overall calorie intake. This can help with weight management and maintaining a healthy body composition.

Lastly, healthy fats can also support the body's metabolic processes. They can help improve insulin sensitivity and regulate blood sugar levels, which can improve the body's ability to burn fat for energy.

It's important to note that while healthy fats can be beneficial for metabolism, they should be consumed in moderation as they are still a source of calories. The recommended daily intake of healthy fats is approximately 20-35% of total daily calorie intake.

fruits and vegetables

High-fibre fruits and vegetables, like broccoli, berries, and leafy greens, are excellent sources of vitamins, minerals, and antioxidants. It aids in lowering the chance of developing chronic illnesses like cancer, diabetes, and heart disease.

Fruits and vegetables play a vital role in our metabolism, which is the process by which our body converts the food we eat into energy. They are rich sources of essential vitamins, minerals, fibre, and other beneficial nutrients that are essential for maintaining optimal health When we consume fruits and vegetables, our body breaks down the carbohydrates, proteins, and fats they contain into glucose, amino acids, and fatty acids. These molecules are then used as fuel to power the body's metabolic processes.

Fruits and vegetables are particularly important because they contain a wide variety of nutrients that are necessary for many of our body's essential functions. For example, they are rich in vitamin C, which is important for immune function and collagen production. They also contain phytochemicals, such as flavonoids and carotenoids, which have antioxidant and anti-inflammatory properties and may help protect against chronic diseases like cancer, heart disease, and diabetes.

Furthermore, fruits and vegetables are rich in fiber, which helps to promote healthy digestion and prevent constipation.

In summary, fruits and vegetables are essential for our metabolism because they provide the nutrients necessary for our body to function properly. Eating a diet rich in fruits and vegetables has been linked to numerous health benefits, including improved immune function, reduced risk of chronic diseases, and better digestive health.

Water

Drinking plenty of water is essential to stay hydrated and support metabolism. Water is involved in many of the body's metabolic processes, including the breakdown and transport of nutrients, and the removal of waste products.

When we don't drink enough water, it can lead to dehydration, which can cause fatigue, headaches, and impair our body's ability to carry out metabolic functions efficiently. Dehydration can also affect our physical and cognitive performance, making it difficult to concentrate or perform physical tasks.

In addition, drinking water can also help to suppress appetite, which can aid in weight loss and weight management. Staying hydrated can also help to reduce fluid retention and bloating.

It's recommended that adults consume at least 8-10 glasses of water per day, or more if they are physically active or live in a hot climate. Other sources of fluids, such as herbal tea, milk, and low-sugar fruit juices, can also contribute to overall hydration.

In summary, staying hydrated with water and other fluids is crucial for supporting metabolism and overall health. Drinking enough water can help to keep our body functioning efficiently, improve physical and cognitive performance, and aid in weight management.

Probiotic-rich foods

Probiotic-rich foods, such as kefir, yoghourt , and sauerkraut, can help promote gut health and support the immune system. They contain beneficial bacteria that can improve digestion and reduce inflammation in the body.

Overall, incorporating these foods into your diet can help improve your health and wellbeing .

They are commonly found in fermented foods and drinks, and can help support a healthy digestive system, boost the immune system, and improve overall health. Some of the probiotics-rich foods that can help boost metabolism include:

- **Yoghourt :** Yoghourt is a popular source of probiotics, containing live cultures of Lactobacillus bulgaricus and Streptococcus thermophilus, which can help boost metabolism and aid in digestion.

- **Kefir:** Kefir is a fermented dairy product that contains live cultures of beneficial bacteria and yeast. It is a good source of probiotics and can help improve gut health and boost metabolism.

- **Sauerkraut:** Sauerkraut is a fermented cabbage dish that is rich in probiotics. It contains Lactobacillus bacteria, which can help improve digestion and boost metabolism.

- **Kimchi:** Kimchi is a spicy Korean dish made from fermented vegetables. It contains live cultures of Lactobacillus bacteria, which can help improve gut health and boost metabolism.

- **Kombucha:** Kombucha is a fermented tea drink that contains live cultures of beneficial bacteria and yeast. It is a good source of probiotics and can help improve gut health and boost metabolism.

- **Miso:** It contains live cultures of beneficial bacteria and can help improve gut health and boost metabolism.

Consuming these probiotics-rich foods on a regular basis can help improve gut health, aid digestion, and boost metabolism, which can lead to better overall health and wellness.

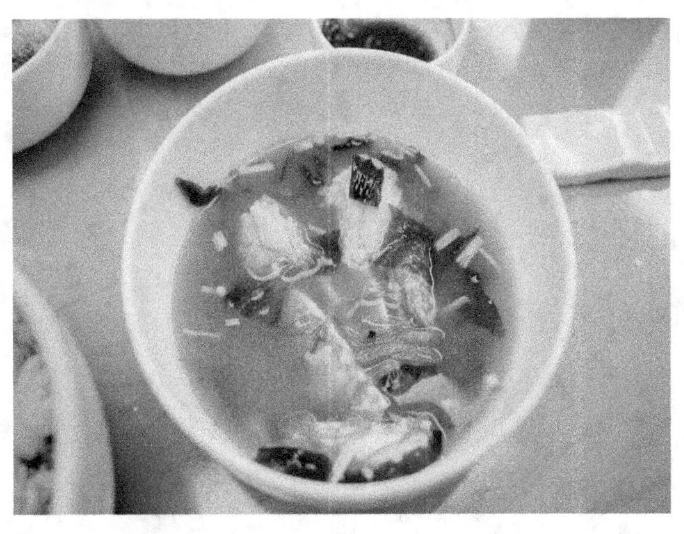

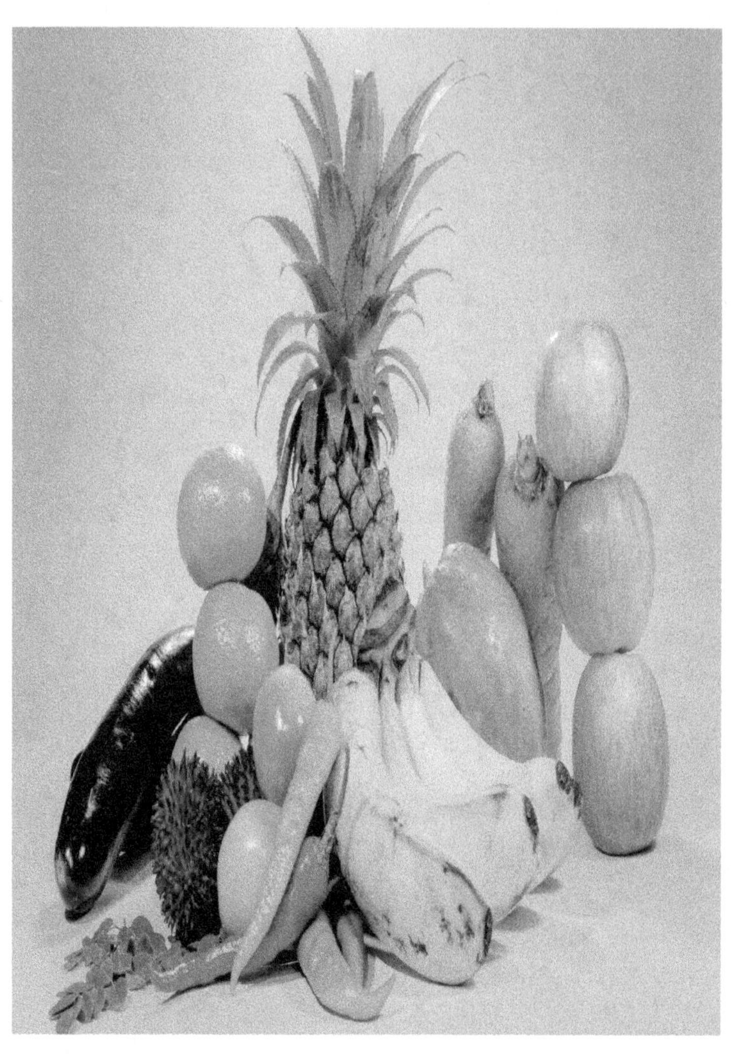

Chapter 3: Foods to Avoid

- Processed foods (chips, cookies, frozen meals)
- Refined sugars (soda, candy, baked goods)
- High glycemic index carbohydrates (white bread, white rice,sugary cereals)
- Trans fats (margarine, fried foods)

In addition to the foods mentioned above , here are a few more to avoid:

1. **Artificial sweeteners:** They may be low in calories, but they can still negatively affect your metabolism and cause cravings for sweet foods.

Here are some examples of artificial sweeteners:

Aspartame(Equal,NutraSweet): This is a low-calorie artificial sweetener made from two amino acids. It is commonly used in diet soft drinks, chewing gum, and sugar-free desserts.

Saccharin (Sweet'N Low):

This is one of the oldest artificial sweeteners and is used in a variety of products including baked goods, jams, and soft drinks.

Sucralose(Splenda):

This sweetener is made from sugar but is modified so that it is calorie-free. It is used in a wide variety of products including baked goods, chewing gum, and soft drinks.

Acesulfame Potassium(Ace-K):

This sweetener is often used in combination with other sweeteners and is found in a variety of products including soft drinks, baked goods, and chewing gum.

Neotame: This sweetener is similar to aspartame but is much sweeter, so less is needed to achieve the desired sweetness. It is used in a variety of products including baked goods and soft drinks.

Advantame: This sweetener is a modified version of aspartame and is used in a variety of products including soft drinks, chewing gum, and baked goods.

It's important to note that while artificial sweeteners are generally considered safe for consumption, some people may experience side effects or have allergic reactions to certain types of sweeteners. As with any food or beverage, it's important to consume artificial sweeteners in moderation as part of a balanced diet.

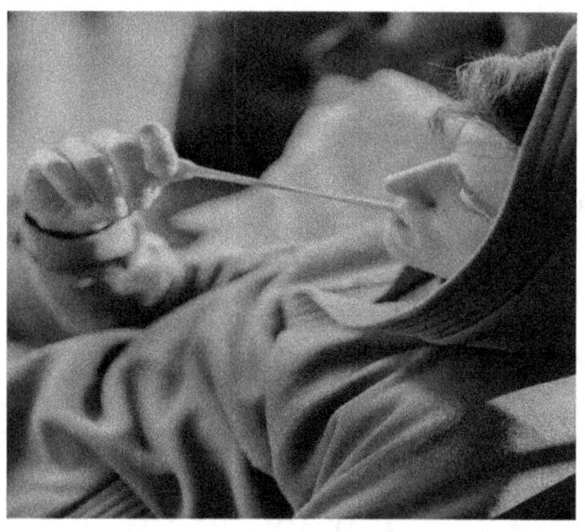

2. **Alcohol:** Drinking too much alcohol can slow down your metabolism and contribute to weight gain.

If you're concerned about your metabolism and want to be mindful of the impact alcohol can have, here is an example of an alcohol to avoid:

Sugary Cocktails: Cocktails that are high in sugar, such as margaritas, piña coladas, or sweetened mixed drinks can cause a spike in your blood sugar levels and may negatively impact your metabolism. The sugar in these drinks can also lead to weight gain over time, which can further slow down your metabolism.

It's important to note that all types of alcohol can have an impact on your metabolism, as alcohol is processed differently by the body than other types of nutrients. Alcohol is metabolised by the liver, and excessive alcohol consumption can cause liver damage and interfere with the body's metabolic processes.

If you choose to drink alcohol, it's important to do so in moderation and to choose drinks that are low in sugar and calories, such as a glass of wine, a light beer, or a vodka soda. Additionally, be sure to stay hydrated and to eat a balanced diet to support your metabolism.

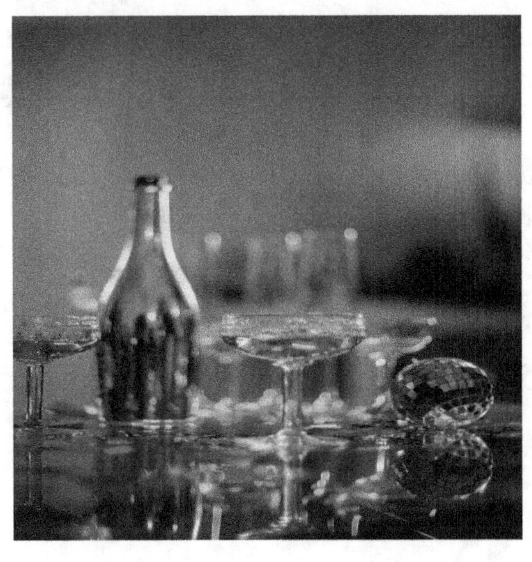

3. **High-fat meats:** Fatty cuts of meat like bacon, sausage, and hot dogs are high in calories and saturated fat, which can negatively impact your metabolism.

Here are some examples of high-fat meats:

Bacon: This is a fatty cut of pork that is often cured and smoked.Due to its high saturated fat content, it should only be eaten occasionally.

Ribeye steak: This is a cut of beef that is known for its marbling and tenderness. While it is flavorful, it is also high in fat and calories.

Sausage: This is a type of ground meat that is often flavoured with herbs and spices. It can be made from pork, beef, or poultry, and is high in fat and calories.

Ground beef (80/20 or higher): This is a common type of beef used in burgers, meatloaf, and other dishes. It is high in fat, especially if it is not lean ground beef.

Chicken thighs with skin: While chicken is a lean protein, chicken thighs with skin are high in fat and calories. Skin removal can aid in lowering the fat level.

It's important to note that consuming high-fat meats in moderation as part of a balanced diet is generally okay for most people. However, excessive consumption of high-fat meats can contribute to weight gain, heart disease, and other health issues. It's recommended to choose lean protein sources, such as chicken breast, turkey, fish, and plant-based proteins, most of the time, and to consume high-fat meats sparingly.

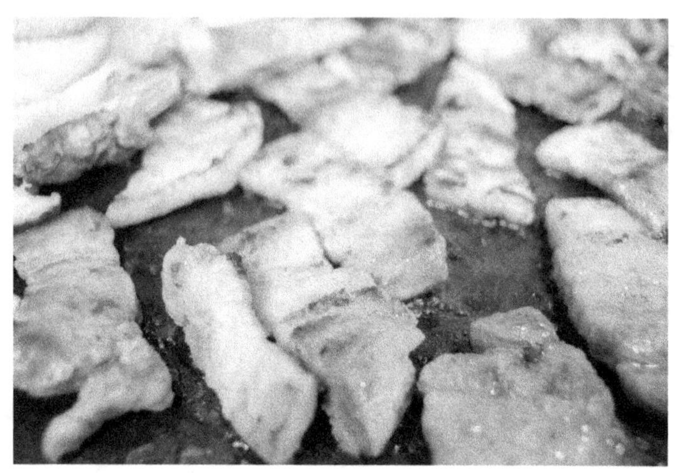

4. **Fried foods**: Fried foods are often cooked in unhealthy oils that can slow down your metabolism and contribute to inflammation.

Fried foods are cooked in hot oil until they are crispy and golden brown. Examples of fried foods include french fries, fried chicken, doughnuts, onion rings, and tempura.

Fried foods are not good for metabolism for several reasons:

High in calories: Fried foods are often high in calories due to the added fat from cooking. This can lead to weight gain and obesity, which can negatively affect metabolism.

High in unhealthy fats: Most fried foods are cooked in oils that are high in unhealthy saturated and trans fats. These fats can increase inflammation in the body, which can impair insulin sensitivity and lead to metabolic disorders like type 2 diabetes.

Reduced nutrient content: The high heat used in frying can destroy or reduce the nutrient content of the food, including vitamins and antioxidants. This can impact metabolism by reducing the body's ability to utilise nutrients effectively.

Can lead to overeating: The crispy texture and savoury flavour of fried foods can make them difficult to resist, leading to overeating. Consuming large amounts of fried foods can disrupt hunger and satiety hormones, leading to a dysregulated metabolism over time.

Overall, consuming fried foods regularly can have negative impacts on metabolism, and it's important to limit their intake in a balanced and healthy diet.

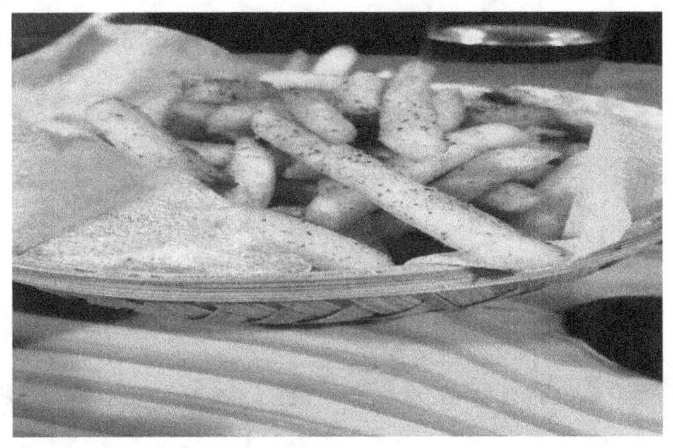

5. High-calorie beverages: High-calorie beverages are drinks that contain a large number of calories, often due to added sugars, sweeteners, or fats. Sodas, energy drinks, and other sugary beverages can add hundreds of calories to your diet without providing any nutritional benefits, leading to weight gain and a slower metabolism.

Here are some examples of high-calorie beverages:

Soda: A can of soda typically contains around 140-150 calories, and many people consume several cans per day.

Sweetened coffee drinks: Beverages like lattes, cappuccinos, and frappuccinos can be loaded with added sugars and syrups, making them high in calories. A typical coffee drink from a coffee shop can contain 300-500 calories.

Fruit juice: Although fruit juice contains vitamins and minerals, it is also high in sugar and calories. A cup of apple juice, for example, can contain around 120-150 calories.

Energy drinks: Energy drinks are often marketed to people who need a quick boost of energy, but they can be very high in calories. A 16-ounce can of an energy drink can contain 200-300 calories.

Alcoholic beverages: Alcoholic beverages can be high in calories due to the alcohol content and added sugars. A glass of wine or beer can contain around 100-200 calories, while cocktails and mixed drinks can have even more.

Remember, a healthy metabolism is key to maintaining a healthy weight and overall well-being. By avoiding these foods and focusing on nutrient-dense whole foods, you can help support your

metabolism and improve your overall
health

Processed foods (chips, cookies, frozen meals)

Processed foods like chips, cookies, and frozen meals often contain high levels of added sugars, unhealthy fats, and artificial ingredients. These ingredients can be harmful to your metabolism in several ways.

Firstly, processed foods often contain refined carbohydrates that can lead to a rapid increase in blood sugar levels. This can cause your body to produce more insulin, which can eventually lead to insulin resistance and type 2 diabetes.

Secondly, processed foods are typically high in unhealthy fats, such as trans fats and saturated fats. These types of fats can increase inflammation in the body and contribute to a variety of health problems, including insulin resistance, obesity, and heart disease.

Finally, processed foods often contain a variety of additives, preservatives, and artificial flavours that can disrupt your gut microbiome, which plays an important role in regulating your metabolism.

To promote a healthy metabolism, it's best to avoid processed foods as much as possible and instead focus on eating a variety of whole, nutrient-dense foods, such as fruits, vegetables, whole grains, lean proteins, and healthy fats. These foods provide your body with the nutrients it needs to function optimally and can help regulate your metabolism in a natural and healthy way.

Refined sugars (soda, candy, baked goods)

Refined sugar, also known as added sugar or processed sugar, can have negative effects on metabolism when consumed in excess. Here are some reasons why:

It can lead to insulin resistance:
When we consume refined sugar, it gets
rapidly absorbed into our bloodstream,
causing a spike in blood sugar levels. This
triggers the release of insulin, a hormone
that helps our cells use glucose for
energy. However, when we consume too
much refined sugar over time, our cells
can become resistant to insulin's effects,
leading to high blood sugar levels and an
increased risk of developing type 2
diabetes.

It can cause inflammation: Studies
have shown that consuming too much
refined sugar can lead to chronic
low-grade inflammation in the body. This
can contribute to a variety of health

problems, including insulin resistance, obesity, and heart disease.

It can disrupt the balance of gut bacteria: Our gut microbiome plays a crucial role in regulating metabolism, and consuming too much refined sugar can disrupt the balance of beneficial and harmful bacteria in our gut. This can lead to digestive problems, inflammation, and an increased risk of developing metabolic disorders.

It can contribute to weight gain: Refined sugar is high in calories but low in nutrients, and consuming too much of it can lead to weight gain and obesity. This, in turn, can increase the risk of developing metabolic syndrome, a cluster of conditions that includes high blood pressure, high blood sugar, and abnormal cholesterol levels.

Overall, while small amounts of refined sugar are unlikely to cause significant harm to most people, consuming too much of it can have negative effects on metabolism and overall health. It's important to limit your intake of refined sugar and focus on a balanced diet that includes plenty of whole, nutrient-dense foods.

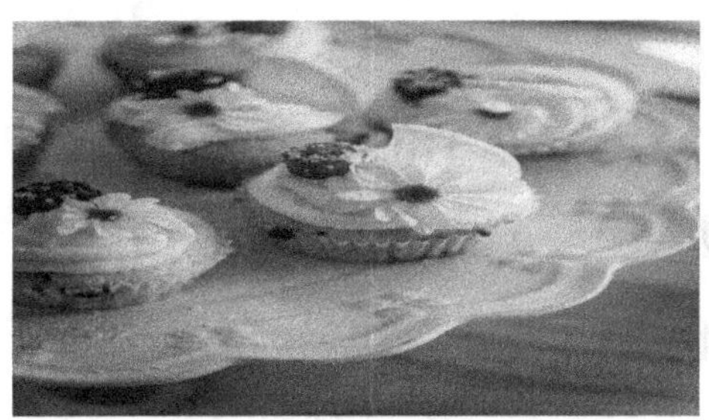

High glycemic index carbohydrates (white bread, white rice, sugary cereals)

High glycemic index carbohydrates are rapidly digested and absorbed by the body, leading to a rapid increase in blood sugar levels. This triggers the release of insulin from the pancreas, which helps to move glucose from the bloodstream into the cells for energy or storage.

However, when large amounts of high glycemic index carbohydrates are consumed, the rapid increase in blood sugar levels can overwhelm the body's ability to produce enough insulin, leading to persistently high blood sugar levels. This can increase the risk of insulin resistance, type 2 diabetes, and other metabolic disorders.

Additionally, high glycemic index carbohydrates can lead to fluctuations in blood sugar levels, which can cause hunger and cravings,

as well as a crash in energy levels after the initial spike.

Therefore, it is recommended to choose carbohydrates with a lower glycemic index, such as whole grains, fruits, vegetables, and legumes, which are digested and absorbed more slowly, leading to a more gradual increase in blood sugar levels and a more sustained release of energy.

Trans fats (margarine, fried foods)

Trans fats are unsaturated fats that have been chemically altered through a process called hydrogenation, which makes them more stable and solid at room temperature. Trans fats can be found in a variety of processed foods, including margarine, fried foods, baked goods, and snack foods.

When consumed, trans fats can be metabolised in the body like any other type of fat. However, trans fats have been shown to have negative effects on metabolism, including raising levels of LDL cholesterol (the "bad" cholesterol) and lowering levels of HDL cholesterol (the "good" cholesterol).

Trans fats have also been shown to increase inflammation in the body, which can contribute to the development of chronic diseases such as heart disease, diabetes, and Alzheimer's disease.

Furthermore, trans fats have been linked to insulin resistance, which can impair the body's ability to use insulin effectively and lead to elevated blood sugar levels. This can increase the risk of developing type 2 diabetes.

Overall, it is recommended to limit or avoid consumption of trans fats as much as possible, and to choose healthier sources of fats such as monounsaturated and polyunsaturated fats found in nuts, seeds, fish, and vegetable oils.

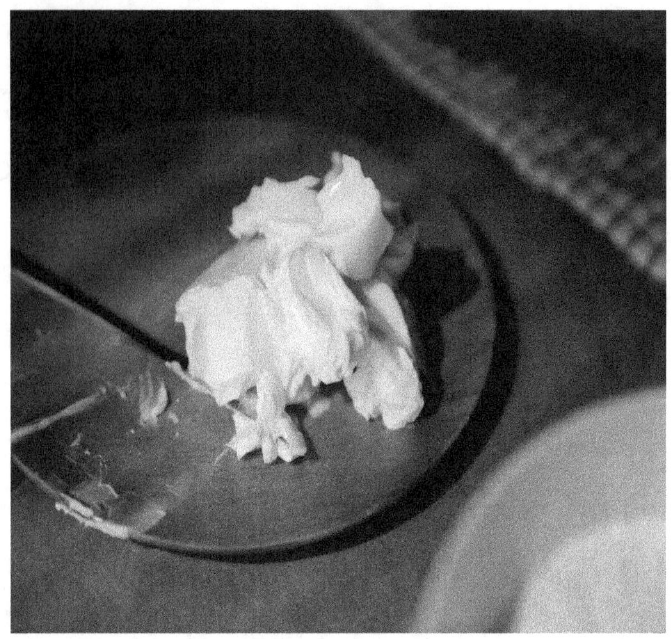

Chapter 4: Meal Plan Examples

Here are some sample breakfast, lunch, and dinner

 recipes that follow the metabolism reset diet:

- **Breakfast:**

feta cheese, greens, and mushrooms in an omelette fruit, chopped nuts, and Greek yoghourt

Almond milk, greens, banana, and chia seeds blended into a smoothie.

- **Lunch:**

Avocado, cherry tomatoes, cucumbers, and mixed vegetables are added to a grilled chicken salad.

Brown rice bowl with grilled salmon and roasted veggies

Whole grain bread served with lentil broth

- **Dinner:**

roasted broccoli and sweet potatoes with baked fish

Brown rice, chicken, and mixed veggies in a stir-fry.

tomato sauce, pork meatballs, and spaghetti squash

- **snacks**

Almond butter spread on apple pieces

yolks that have been hard boiled

sliced banana, honey, and roasted legumes in Greek yoghourt

Baby carrots and chopped bell peppers in hummus

Trail blend with dried fruit and mixed nuts

These snacks and dinners are composed of lean protein, healthy fats, and fibre-rich carbohydrates to help speed up metabolism and keep you feeling full and satiated all day.

The above-mentioned meal plan examples are created to adhere to the ideals of a diet that increases metabolism and includes a balance of lean protein, healthy fats, and fibre-rich carbohydrates.

Protein, good fats, and fibre are available in morning foods like omelettes with spinach and feta, Greek yoghurt with berries and nuts, and smoothies made with chia seeds and almond milk.

Lunch choices include lentil soup with whole grain bread, brown rice bowls with salmon and roasted vegetables, and grilled chicken salad with vegetables and avocado. To help you feel satisfied and energised, these choices offer a balance of protein, fibre, and healthy carbohydrates.

Dinner choices include stir-fry with chicken and mixed vegetables, baked salmon with sweet potatoes and broccoli, and spaghetti squash, turkey meatballs, and tomato sauce offer a satisfying combination of fibre-rich carbs, lean protein, and good fats.

Last but not least, a variety of snacks, including apple slices with almond butter, hard-boiled eggs, roasted chickpeas, Greek yoghourt with honey and sliced banana, hummus with baby carrots and sliced bell peppers, and mixed nuts and dried fruit trail mix, offer a combination of protein, healthy fats, and fibre to help speed up metabolism and keep you feeling full in between meals.

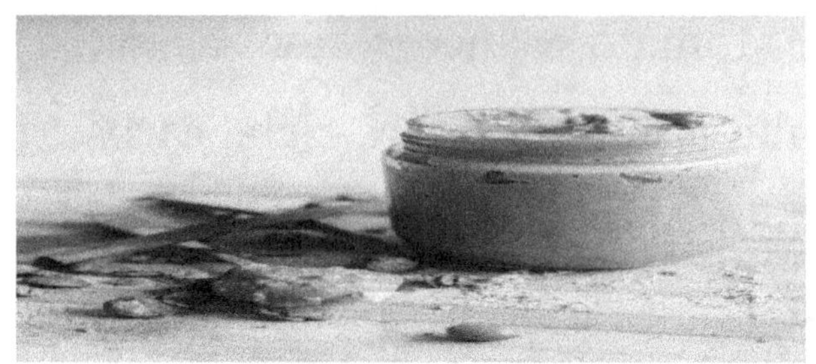

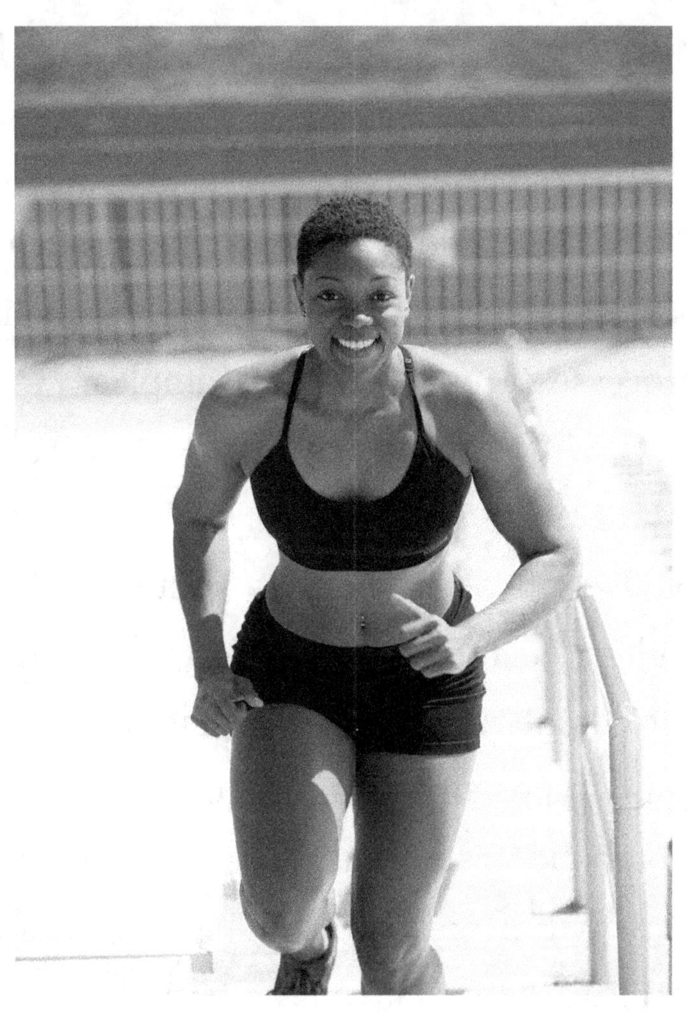

Chapter 5: Recommended exercises

There are a number of exercises that can be beneficial for improving metabolic processes. Here are some examples:

1.High-Intensity Interval Training (HIIT):

HIIT involves short bursts of high-intensity exercise followed by brief periods of rest or low-intensity exercise. This type of training can increase metabolic rate and improve insulin sensitivity.Here's are some example of a HIIT workout that you can try:

Warm-up: Start with a 5-10 minute light cardio warm-up, such as jogging, jumping jacks, or cycling.

Sprint intervals: Sprint at maximum effort for 20 seconds, followed by 10 seconds of rest. Repeat this pattern for a total of 8 rounds, which will take 4 minutes.

Recovery: Take a 2-3 minute break to recover and catch your breath.

Burpee intervals: Perform burpees at maximum effort for 20 seconds, followed by 10 seconds of rest. Repeat this pattern for a total of 8 rounds, which will take 4 minutes.

Recovery: Take another 2-3 minute break to recover and catch your breath.

Jump rope intervals: Jump rope at maximum effort for 20 seconds, followed by 10 seconds of rest. Repeat this pattern for a total of 8 rounds, which will take 4 minutes.

Cool-down: Finish with a 5-10 minute light cardio cool-down, such as walking, stretching, or yoga.

This workout will take about 20-30 minutes and can be adjusted based on your fitness level and preferences. Remember to always listen to your body and modify or take breaks as needed.

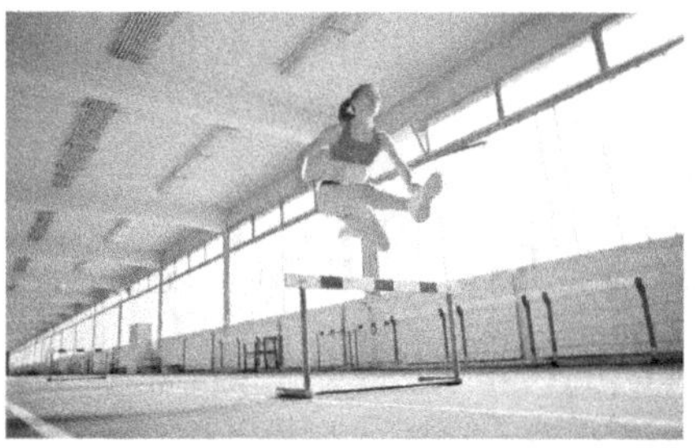

2.Resistance Training:

Resistance training, such as weight lifting, can help increase muscle mass and improve metabolic rate. As muscle tissue requires more energy to maintain than fat tissue, having more muscle can help increase overall energy expenditure. It is also known as strength training, involves exercises that use resistance to build muscle strength, endurance, and size. Here are some examples of resistance training exercises:

Weightlifting: This involves lifting weights, such as dumbbells, barbells, or kettlebells, to perform exercises such as:

1. Bicep curls
2. Squat
3. Bench presses.

Bodyweight exercises: These exercises use your body weight as resistance, such as:

1. Push-ups

2. Pull-ups

3. Squats.

Resistance bands: These elastic bands provide resistance when stretched, and can be used for exercises such as

bicep curls

tricep extensions

leg lifts.

Suspension training: This involves using a suspension trainer, such as a TRX, to perform exercises that use your own body weight as resistance.

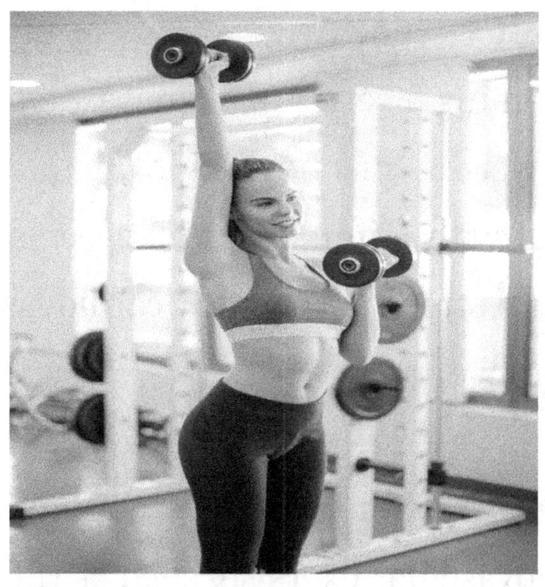

Isometric exercises: These exercises involve holding a position for a set amount of time, such as a plank or wall sit.

Plyometrics: These explosive exercises involve jumping, hopping, or bounding to build power and strength, such as jump squats or box jumps.

Circuit training: This involves performing a series of exercises, typically with weights or bodyweight , in a circuit format with minimal rest between sets to build strength and cardiovascular endurance.

3.Cardiovascular Exercise:

Cardiovascular exercise, such as running, cycling, or swimming, can improve cardiovascular health and increase metabolic rate. This type of exercise can also improve insulin sensitivity and help regulate blood sugar levels.

There are various types of cardiovascular exercises, which are also referred to as aerobic exercises, that can be performed to improve cardiovascular endurance and overall fitness. Here are some examples of cardiovascular exercises:

- Running
- Walking
- Cycling
- Swimming
- Rowing
- Jumping rope
- High-intensity interval training (HIIT)
- Dancing
- Kickboxing
- Cross-country skiing
- Elliptical machine workouts
- Stair climbing

- Aerobic classes (such as step aerobics, Zumba, or dance fitness)
- Circuit training
- Hiking

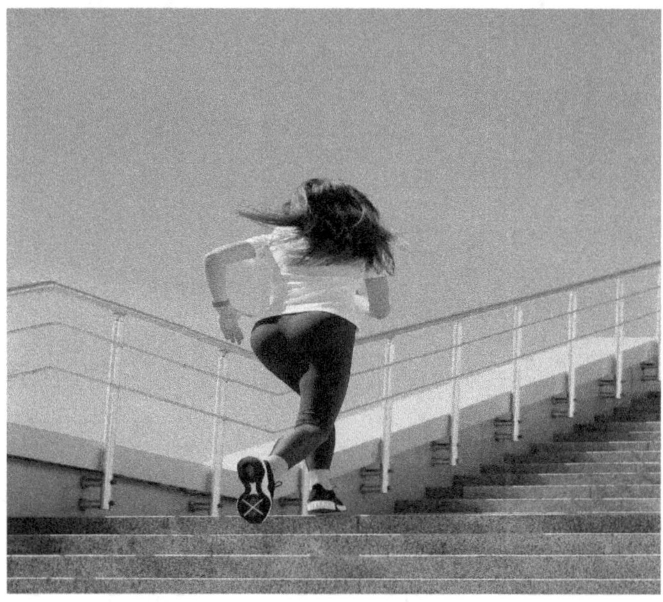

It's important to choose a form of cardiovascular exercise that you enjoy and that fits your fitness level and goals. Aim to get at least 150 minutes of moderate-intensity cardio exercise or 75 minutes of high-intensity cardio exercise per week to improve cardiovascular health and overall fitness.

4.Circuit Training:

Circuit training involves completing a series of exercises in a sequence with little to no rest in between. This type of training can help increase metabolic rate and improve overall fitness.Circuit training is a form of exercise that involves performing a series of exercises in a specific order, with little to no rest in between. This type of workout can help to improve cardiovascular endurance, build strength, and burn calories. Here are some examples of circuit training exercises that can be combined to create a full-body workout:

- Jumping jacks
- Squats
- Push-ups
- Lunges
- Burpees
- Plank
- Mountain climbers
- High knees
- Tricep dips
- Sit-ups
- Box jumps
- Kettlebell swings
- Battle rope waves
- Medicine ball slams

- Jump rope

To perform circuit training, choose 5-10 exercises and perform each one for a set amount of time (e.g., 30-60 seconds) or a set number of repetitions (e.g., 10-15 reps). Take a short rest period (e.g., 10-30 seconds) in between each exercise and complete the circuit 2-3 times for a full workout. Circuit training can be done with bodyweight exercises or with equipment like dumbbells, resistance bands, or medicine balls. It's important to choose exercises that target different muscle groups to ensure a full-body workout.

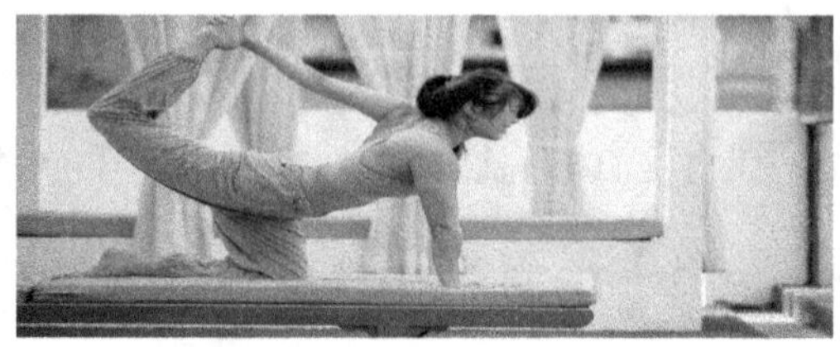

5.Yoga: Although yoga may not be a traditional form of exercise for increasing metabolic rate, it can still have a positive impact on metabolism. Certain yoga poses can help increase muscle strength, improve flexibility, and reduce stress levels, all of which can improve metabolic function.

There are many different styles of yoga, each with their own unique postures (asanas) and breathing techniques (pranayama). Here are some examples:

- **Hatha Yoga:** This is a gentle form of yoga that involves holding poses for several breaths and focusing on breathing and relaxation.

- **Vinyasa Yoga:** This is a more dynamic form of yoga that involves flowing through a series of poses with each movement linked to the breath.

- **Ashtanga Yoga:** This is a more physically demanding form of yoga that involves a set sequence of postures that are performed in a specific order.

- **Bikram Yoga:** Also known as hot yoga, this style involves practising yoga in a heated room, which can help increase flexibility and detoxify the body.

- **Restorative Yoga:** This is a deeply relaxing form of yoga that involves holding gentle poses for an extended period of time, often with the support of props such as blankets and bolsters.

- **Yin Yoga:** This is a slower form of yoga that involves holding passive stretches for several minutes to release tension in the body and increase flexibility.

- **Kundalini Yoga:** This form of yoga emphasises the connection between the mind, body, and spirit, and involves practising specific poses, breathing techniques, and

meditation to awaken the kundalini
energy in the body.

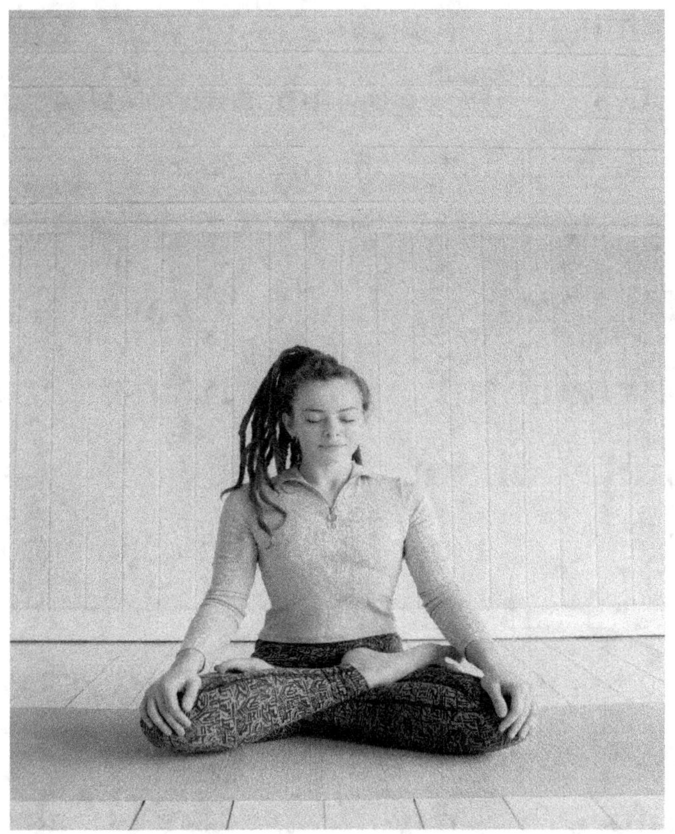

It is important to note that the most
effective exercise program will be one
that includes a variety of exercises and is

tailored to an individual's specific needs and fitness level. Additionally, maintaining a balanced diet and staying hydrated are also important factors in improving metabolic processes.

Why you should take exercise serious for a good health and metabolism

Exercise is crucial for maintaining good health and a healthy metabolism. Here are some reasons why you should take exercise seriously:

Improves cardiovascular health: Regular exercise can strengthen your heart and lungs, improve blood circulation, and reduce the risk of heart disease.

Helps keep a healthy weight: Exercise can aid in calorie burning and weight maintenance. Numerous health issues, such as high blood pressure, diabetes, and heart disease, can be brought on by being overweight or fat.

Boosts metabolism: Regular exercise can boost your metabolism, which helps your body burn calories
more efficiently even when you're not exercising.

Reduces the risk of chronic diseases: Exercise can help reduce the risk of many chronic diseases, including type 2 diabetes, stroke, and some types of cancer.

Enhances mental health: Exercise is known to reduce symptoms of depression and anxiety, and can improve your overall mood and sense of well-being.

Builds strength and flexibility: Exercise can help build muscle mass, increase bone density, and improve flexibility and balance.

Promotes better sleep: Regular exercise can help you fall asleep faster, sleep more deeply, and wake up feeling more refreshed.

In summary, regular exercise is essential for maintaining good health and a healthy metabolism. It can improve cardiovascular health, help maintain a healthy weight, boost metabolism, reduce the risk of chronic diseases, enhance mental health, build strength and flexibility, and promote better sleep.

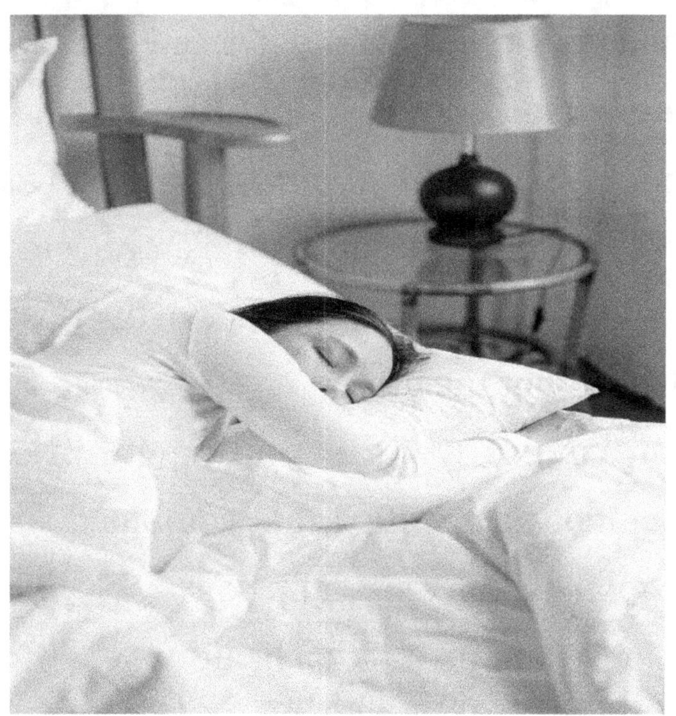

Chapter 6: Lifestyle Changes

You can experience a number of advantages when you adopt healthy living habits and adhere to a metabolism-correcting diet, including:

Increased energy levels: A healthy metabolism allows your body to convert food into energy more efficiently, which can help you feel more energised throughout the day.

Improved weight management: A metabolism rectified diet combined with regular exercise can help you
achieve and maintain a healthy weight.

Reduced risk of chronic diseases: A healthy diet and lifestyle can help to reduce your risk of chronic diseases such as heart disease, diabetes, and certain types of cancer.

Improved digestion: A metabolism rectified diet that is rich in fibre and nutrients can help to improve digestion and reduce gastrointestinal problems such as bloating and constipation.

Better mood and mental health: A healthy lifestyle can positively impact your mood and mental health by reducing stress levels, improving sleep quality, and increasing overall feelings of well-being.

Remember, everyone's body is different, and results may vary depending on your individual circumstances. It's important to consult with a healthcare professional before making any major changes to your diet or exercise routine.

The importance of regular exercise and physical activity for boosting metabolism

Regular exercise and physical activity are crucial for boosting metabolism, which is the process by which the body converts food into energy. When you exercise, you increase the amount of energy your body uses, which can help to increase your metabolism over time.

One of the main ways exercise boosts metabolism is by increasing muscle mass. Muscle is more metabolically active than fat, which means that it burns more calories at rest. When you engage in regular exercise that includes strength training, you can build and maintain muscle mass, which helps to increase your metabolism.

In addition to building muscle mass, exercise can also increase the number of mitochondria in your cells. Mitochondria are responsible for producing energy in the body, and the more mitochondria you have, the more energy your body can produce. This, in turn, can help to boost your metabolism and make it easier for your body to burn calories.

Other ways that regular exercise can boost metabolism include:

Increasing heart rate and breathing rate, which can help to burn more calories and increase energy expenditure

Reducing insulin resistance, which can help to improve the body's ability to use glucose for energy Increasing levels of certain hormones, such as growth hormone and testosterone, which can help to increase muscle mass and metabolism

Overall, regular exercise and physical activity are important for maintaining a healthy metabolism and promoting weight loss or weight management. It's recommended to aim for at least 150 minutes of moderate-intensity exercise or 75 minutes of vigorous-intensity exercise per week, in addition to incorporating strength training exercises at least two days per week.

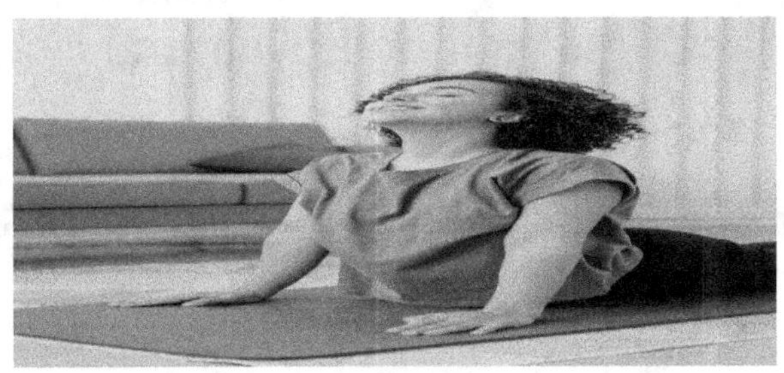

Tips for getting enough sleep and managing stress, both of which can affect metabolism

The two most important things for keeping a good metabolism are getting enough sleep and controlling stress. Here are some pointers for getting more rest and reducing stress:

- **Maintain a regular sleep schedule**: Even on weekends, try to go to bed and rise up at the same times every day. This enhances the quality of your sleep and serves to regulate your body's natural clock.

- **Establish a peaceful sleeping environment**: Maintain a cool, quiet, and dark bedroom to encourage unwinding and sound slumber. Think about making an investment in soft linens, cushions, and a sturdy mattress.

- **Prioritise sleep over computer time**: Your body's normal sleep-wake cycle can be hampered by exposure to blue light from electronic devices. At least an hour before going to bed, put away your phone, computer, and device.

- **Utilise calming methods**: Effective methods for lowering tension and fostering relaxation include yoga, meditation, deep breathing, and progressive muscle relaxation.

- **Keep moving**: Regular exercise can help to reduce stress and enhance the quality of sleep. Try to exercise for at least 30 minutes, most days of the week, at a moderate effort.

- Seek assistance Discuss any potential stressors with peers, family, or a mental health professional. You can better manage your stress by having a support structure.

- **Avoid drinking alcohol and caffeine:** They both interfere with slumber and raise stress levels. Avoid using these substances entirely or only in moderation, particularly in the evening.

- **Sleep**

You can enhance your general health and increase your metabolism by changing your sleeping patterns and stress-reduction methods.

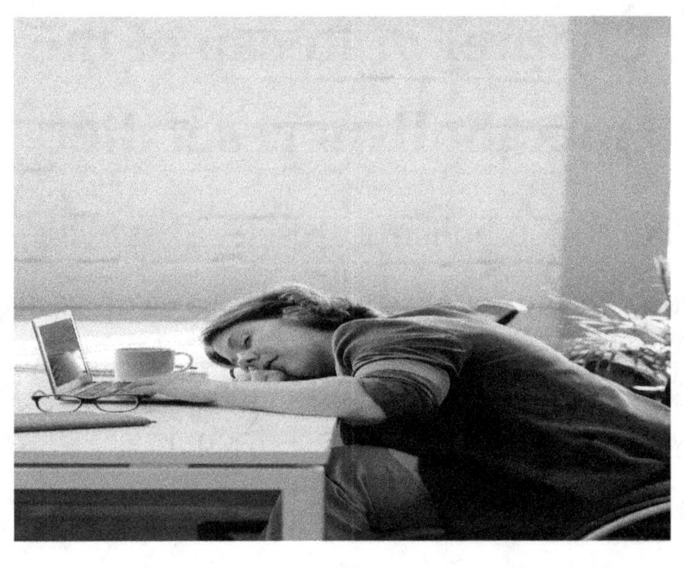

Chapter 7: Recap of the metabolism reset diet

The metabolism reset diet is a comprehensive approach to improving your metabolic health and overall well-being. By focusing on nutrient-dense whole foods, balancing macronutrient intake, and incorporating intermittent fasting, this diet can help you achieve sustainable weight loss, increased energy, and better metabolic function.

Some of the benefits of the metabolism reset diet include improved insulin sensitivity, lower inflammation, improved cognitive function, and reduced risk of chronic diseases like type 2 diabetes and cardiovascular disease.

While the metabolism reset diet can provide significant short-term benefits, it's important to remember that sustainable lifestyle changes are crucial for long-term success. It's essential to incorporate regular exercise, stress management techniques, and mindfulness practices into your daily routine to support your overall health and well-being.

In summary, the metabolism reset diet can be an effective tool for improving your metabolic health and overall wellness. However, it's important to approach any dietary change with a long-term perspective and a commitment to sustainable lifestyle habits.

Benefits and encouragement to make sustainable lifestyle changes for the long-term.

Making sustainable lifestyle changes can be challenging, but with determination and commitment, it is possible to achieve long-term success. Here are some encouraging tips to help you make sustainable lifestyle changes:

Start small: Don't try to make drastic changes all at once. Instead, focus on making small changes that you can maintain over time. For example, start by drinking more water, eating more fruits and vegetables, or taking the stairs instead of the elevator.

Set realistic goals: It's important to set goals that are achievable and realistic.By pursuing excellence, you'll only set yourself up for failure.Instead, aim for progress and celebrate your small victories along the way.

Find a support system: Having a support system can make all the difference in the world when it comes to making sustainable lifestyle changes. Consider joining a group or finding a friend who shares similar goals and can offer encouragement and accountability.

Be mindful of your habits: Pay attention to the habits that are keeping you from living a sustainable lifestyle. For example, if you tend to eat junk food when you're stressed, try finding a healthier way to cope with stress such as exercise or meditation.

Educate yourself: Learning about the benefits of a sustainable lifestyle can be motivating and empowering. Read books, watch documentaries, or attend workshops that focus on sustainable living.

As for metabolism and diet, it's important to remember that everyone's body is different and what works for one person may not work for another. A balanced diet that includes a variety of whole foods is a good place to start.For individualised advice, speak with a certified dietitian or other healthcare provider.

Summary /Conclusion

To boost diet and support weight loss, it's important to focus on a balanced diet that includes nutrient-rich foods and avoids excess calories from added sugars and unhealthy fats. Here are some tips to support weight loss:

Put an emphasis on whole, nutritious foods: Include a lot of fresh produce in your diet, along with whole grains, lean meats, and healthy fats.

Avoid processed and high-calorie foods: Limit your intake of processed and high-calorie foods, such as fast food, sugary drinks, and packaged snacks.

Watch portion sizes: Pay attention to your portion sizes and try to avoid overeating.

Stay hydrated: Drink plenty of water and avoid sugary drinks and alcohol.

Incorporate physical activity: Regular exercise can help boost metabolism and support weight loss.

Get enough sleep: Aim for 7-9 hours of sleep per night, as sleep deprivation can disrupt metabolism and lead to weight gain.

Weight loss is a gradual process and there are no quick fixes. It's important to focus on making sustainable lifestyle changes rather than relying on fad diets or extreme measures. To create a customised strategy that is effective for you, speak with a certified dietitian or other healthcare professional.

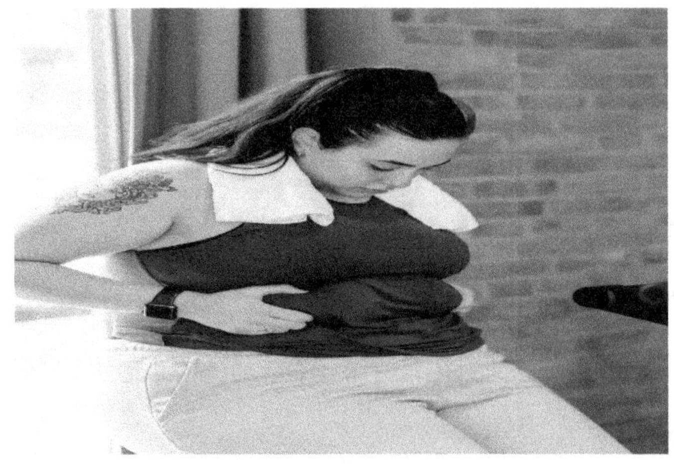

Remember that making sustainable changes to your diet and lifestyle takes time and patience, but the long-term benefits are worth it.